Detoxifying your body

Ilary P. Kopp

Copyright © 2022 by Ilary P. Kopp

All rights reserved.

No portion of this book may be reproduced in any form without written permission from the publisher or author, except as permitted by U.S. copyright law.

Contents

1. Introduction 1
2. The circular system 21
3. The million 51
4. For my liver 84
5. Hepatic plant 99
6. Workouts 117

Chapter One

Introduction

Liver health is important. Lately my stomach has risen. Many foods cause stomach pain and it lasts for some time. I have had stomach problems and headaches lately and I feel a bit lethargic. I often feel tired and weak. I also suffer from acne and am often constipated. STOP! How long will you endure these hardships? Your liver is overloaded and you may think that these symptoms are inevitable and there is nothing you can do about it. You can rejuvenate your liver by cleansing, detoxifying and removing all residues, fats and toxins that overload it. You will be able to get rid of all these annoying problems and thus restore your health and strength. To stay healthy, all the organs of the body must function properly. While each organ is important because a deficiency in any of these organs can have a devastating effect on the entire body, the liver is especially important because it allows the other organs to do their jobs. The liver is a complex organ. It is the body's first line of defense against foreign toxins and poisons, making it the body's most important defender and protector. Due to the inability to process waste, the body's cells become overwhelmed with toxic waste. Because our body is attacked and unable to function properly, the starting point for most of our diseases, according to naturopathy, is the accumulation of these dangerous chemicals. Today, a society that encourages overeating, overeating, and overeating is rampant. Air, water, insecticides in food and harmful compounds in everyday products are all sources of environmental pollution that are almost impossible to avoid. Obstruction of the liver is caused by all these factors that put a lot of pressure on the liver. Liver toxicity may be directly related to the increase in cardiovascular, allergic, or immune diseases that we see more and more today. To protect the body, we need to help the liver and cleanse it so that we can regenerate it.Liver disease is a fact of life for most people. Although this book is written for people with digestive diseases related to the liver, it is important for those who suffer from other diseases and those who understand the important role of the liver in restoring health.Part of this book introduces the concept of detoxification and how it can help restore your health in terms such as perspective, toxins, excretory organs, and drainage. Knowing more about liver function will help you understand its importance. If the liver does not function properly, it can lead to many health problems. The main treatment for liver failure is detoxification, as the organ is clogged with toxins. In the second half of the book, you will learn how to quickly, easily and effectively detoxify your body. Auxiliary home remedies and medications are listed at the end of this section. Although they are easily observable, you should always seek the advice of a doctor if you have any concerns or questions. Introduction to liver functionWhat is the detoxification point of the liver?Naturopathy is very important to cleanse the whole body, especially the liver. Describing the natural landscape - the cellular environment of the body - helps to better understand the therapeutic effectiveness of these treatments.? is it rightNaturopathy is a unique branch of noninvasive primary care that uses medications and techniques that stimulate the body's natural ability to heal.

Concept of landscapeYour organs and tissues consist of a collection of cells. Every organism has a cell. Within each cell is a group of specialized structures called organelles, each of which has a unique function for the cell or organism. Ultimately, these activities allow the body to breathe, produce energy, eliminate waste, and reproduce. ? is it right The basic cell model is the same for everyone, although their purpose varies from cell to cell. Many cell types in the body can be detected by this system, including the kidneys, liver, colon, bones, muscles, and nerves. Cells, like all living things, can grow only under the right conditions. This liquid habitat makes up 70% of our body mass and is known as the human body surface. There are many kinds of liquids on Earth. Direct contact between some of these fluids and cells: The name "intracellular fluid" is explained by the fact that it fills the cells inside. This fluid, which makes up half of our weight, is the basis of our body structure. Unlike intracellular fluid, interstitial or extracellular fluid is outside the cells. Cells bathe and are surrounded by it. Extracellular fluid makes up 15% of our body mass and is the external environment of the cell. Cells are not in direct contact with other terrestrial fluids:• Blood vessels carry blood through the body. Lymph vessels carry lymph. These two fluids make up 5% of our body weight.? is it rightSuch mineral salts as calcium, magnesium and potassium make up only 30% of the total weight of the human body. Bones, skulls, hair and tendons contain very hard particles. In addition, mineral salts are necessary for the structure of cell membranes, tissues and organs. The survival of the cell depends entirely on the environment in which it is located, so the composition of these physiological fluids is important.Excellent level For physical health, the landscape must have the right composition to support cells and organs with maximum vigor and endurance. The main consequence of this ideal scenario is that if you change this composition, your health and well-being will suffer. * 1The cellular landscape of the organism is often changed to a favorable state by the addition of chemicals. Guidelines for these compounds include urate acid, urea, and other substances not normally found in the landscape, although present in moderate amounts (contaminants, food additives, etc.). According to naturopathy, the accumulation of these toxins is the root cause of disease. These toxins must be removed from the body in order to heal. The lack of necessary chemicals can also affect the composition of the landscape. For example, we can mention vitamins, minerals and rare elements that are normally present in the soil, but for some reason are not present in sufficient quantities. Malnutrition is the main cause of this problem and can be corrected by providing the body with the nutrients it lacks through diet or supplements.Why do we get sick from toxins?Drunkenness of the body can cause various health problems. The blood thickens, making it difficult for it to pass through the arteries of the circulatory system. Lymph and other cellular fluids are tubes for waste that would otherwise be transported to the excretory organs by the bloodstream. If this situation persists, the fluids become heavily contaminated and blocked.Cells are absorbed by an inert substance and disrupt any binding. Without oxygen and nutrients, cells and the organs they form cannot perform their functions.

When debris accumulates, the body's ability to function effectively is impaired. As debris accumulates in the walls of blood vessels, blood flow decreases, and the amount of water exchanged between tissues decreases. This causes stiffness in the joints, blockage of the kidneys, closure of the skin and congestion in the liver. Rubbish irritates the tissues and mucous membranes of the body. Their inflammation later leads to their hardness and sclerosis. In addition, they are more susceptible to infection. The beginning of the change of cancer cells Poisons cause damage for the following reasons: Their weight, as they take up a lot of space, blocks and blocks the flow of cells and blood vessels. • Their prejudice. Inflamed cells die due to their inflammatory effect. Toxic overload causes disease If the cause of the disease is toxins, they can be clearly identified. This is a fair decision. Accumulation of toxins does not disable the body. Instead, he takes steps to get rid of them. And the presence of toxins and the body's efforts to eliminate toxins are factors that cause disease. Preventing and coughing is often responsible for respiratory disorders such as asthma, bronchitis, colds or sinusitis, as they are our alveoli, bronchial and bronchitis, throat, claw and nose (common cold (common cold (overall cold).In all skin complications, acidic ingredients (dry eczema, cracks and disconnected skin) or pulp waste (sebaceous glands) are discarded (acne, boiling, oily skin, eczema). Insufficiency, indigestion, nausea, vomiting and diarrhea are symptoms of overeating in your system. If irritated or fermenting chemicals cause gastritis, enteritis or colitis in the digestive tract, if they irritate or ferment mucous membranes (inflammation). WARNING!Indole, phenol, hydrogen sulfide, methane and phthamine are toxic and irritating chemicals produced by fermentation and putrefaction in the intestine. Inflamed, narrow and uncomfortable joints can get worse if left untreated (paralysis). Urgic acid crystals can grow in organs or tissues around, causing inflammation and tissue damage during part of arthritis.Blood thickening, shrinking in the arteries and thickening of their walls (arterial colitis) and the presence of cardiovascular disorders (fat, fatty acids) that cause cardiovascular disorders that can distort or prevent nerves (attacks (heart attack , stroke. Kidney disease is caused by protein waste. Excess fat causes obesity. Sugar is the leading cause of diabetes. Both carcinogens and allergens cause cancer. Stomach acid is the leading cause of stomach ulcers.Tox ins and waste are produced and eliminated in a symbiotic relationship. Exclusive interview with Robert Mason, founder of XenaWhere exactly do toxins come from?One source of these toxins are toxins that accumulate in the body as a result of tissue damage. All depleted cells and dead red blood cells must be permanently removed from the body. Most toxins are produced in the body by food. Proteins, carbohydrates and lipids produce uric acid and urea, as well as lactic acid and various other acids.These toxins are regularly produced in the body and eliminated by the system. However, when a person eats too much, the concentration of toxins is abnormally high. As a result, in industrialized civilizations, frequent overeating causes the body to accumulate toxic waste that the system can no longer eliminate. As a result, substances that cannot be removed from the body accumulate in the cellular lan dscape.Toxic substances: what is the issue? On the other hand, toxic chemicals should not remain in the body. Poisonous chemicals disrupt the normal functioning of the body and affect the whole body. These include all chemical toxins released from air, water, or soil pollution (such as lead, cadmium, and mercury).Chemicals used in industrial agriculture to treat food and animals are important sources of exposure to hazardous foreign chemicals, including many insecticides, herbicides, and fungicides. The American Cancer Society estimates that at least 70 of the more than 4,000 chemicals in tobacco smoke, such as benzene, uranium, and formaldehyde, are carcinogenic, and many others cause serious health problems. Toxic chemicals are also found in many medications and vaccines. It is difficult to remove them because the human body is unable to absorb or remove them. The liver, with its cleansing power, perfectly neutralizes and removes them. Toxins and toxins that are organized according to the entrance pointThere are three main ways to enter the body of toxins and harmful chemicals.Consumption of food and drinkInappropriate consumption of products such as sugar (as well as fat, protein and saltTypes of ingredients to improve the taste, color or layer of foodUse of weeds, pesticides and mushrooms in agricultureAntibiotics, growth increases and other drugs used in agriculture on animals• drugs and drugs• Water and products are contaminatedCirculatory systemMassive polluted air (industrial emissions, cars emissions, etc.)Air with high concentration of particlesDue to the effects of smoking,

other personal hygiene products and cosmetics made of synthetic and organic materials; talc and other powders; worms; hair color; shampoo; deodorant; hair conditioner; to worry;? is it right Excessive food not only increases body weight, but also causes the accumulation of toxins in the body. If you have too much toxic waste in your body, you will not gain weight. Excretion of toxins: organs of excretion. 'To maintain a clean physiological cellular landscape, the body has five organs that remove toxins from the blood and expel them from the body. Examples of these organs are the liver, intestines, kidneys, skin and lungs. These secretory organs, called immune organs, are responsible for removing toxins from the body and ensuring their removal. When these organs function properly, toxins are not produced or consumed in large quantities, and the environment becomes clean. Because the excretory organs remove toxins as quickly as they enter the body, cells can function normally.

DETOXIFYING YOUR BODY

Basic elementsToxins that are too much for the organs to remove quickly outweigh their ability to remove them, and more toxins begin to accumulate in the landscape. Too much accumulation of toxins when the organs of excretion are sluggish or weak can lead to disease. Removes toxins from the bodyOnly the accumulation of toxins in the body can cause disease, so the best treatment is to try to get rid of these toxins from the body. Drainage or cleansing, often referred to today as detoxification, is a method used to achieve this goal of removing toxins. * 2Because the body's excretory systems are stimulated during cleansing, circulating toxins are filtered and removed from the body more quickly.Trainers - food, herbs, massage and hydrotherapy - can be used to stimulate the organ system and increase the ability to remove the boil. Boiling organs are the body's main mechanism for removing toxins.

All procedures aimed at improving the cleansing process of the body are concentrated on these elements. The purpose of treatment is to restore the normal rate of secretion or, more precisely, to temporarily increase it to compensate for the delay in secretion. During the drainage procedure, the ejaculate organs are strongly activated, leading to increased secretion of slag products. As a result of this increased deletion, it should be clear:• The intestine passes more material, or intestines become more frequent. The garbage in the urine becomes charged and darker as the volume of urine increases. An increase in skin temperature leads to an increase in sweat.• Colloidal debris deposited in the respiratory tract is secreted. As a result of the treatment, the level of toxins in the tissues decreases. When the cell landscape returns to its original state, the symptoms of the disease diminish and then disappear.

By removing toxins from the body, the organs can restore their desired function. The internal capacity of the organ for repair and the extent of damage already caused by these injuries affect the likelihood of regeneration. The main properties of the liverAll five excretory organs are located in the human digestive system. The liver is not more important for a healthy body than the other four organs, but as we will see, it occupies a unique place in the body. Like any other excretory system, toxins are eliminated from the body by the liver. However, it removes toxins and neutralizes them. Only the ureters and ureters have this ability, not as much as the other four. A very small percentage of them can neutralize toxic substances. WARNING!Despite its main function of removing toxins and toxic chemicals, the liver becomes blocked and cannot function normally.As a result, the liver is one of the organs of excretion that must be kept in perfect condition. If a patient requires an excretory organ due to impaired physiological function, the liver is usually the most appropriate choice. Toxins and toxic chemicals put a lot of pressure on the liver and the liver cannot handle it. In this case, the first priority is to detoxify the liver to avoid endangering other parts of the body.Restart• Toxins are the leading cause of disease. • The liver is one of the main organs for removing toxins.Toxins and toxic chemicals are neutralized by the liver. Anatomy of the liverThe liver plays an important role in the metabolism of our body.Sandra Cabot, Medical Director, Australian Women's Health Advisory ServiceTo properly care for the liver, you need to have a complete knowledge of it. What does it look like in real life? In what part of the body is it located and how does it interact with other organs?

20   DETOXIFYING YOUR BODY

Chapter Two

The circular system

The portal vein, hepatic artery, and hepatic vein connect the liver to the rest of the body. The liver receives blood from two of these veins, and a third vein returns it to the rest of the body. ? is it right As for blood vessels, "like the size of thin hair" is a common word for capillaries (Latin: recording). As a result, capillaries are seven times thin than hair. The vein is connected to the portal veinThe portal vein, which is formed by the capillaries of the intestinal wall, supplies 75% of the blood to the liver. Microtubes absorb nutrients from food in the digestive tract. The mucous membrane of the toxic corrupt intestine increases the penetration of capillaries, which allows dangerous food compounds to absorb blood flow. Blood flowing through the portal nerve has different cases depending on the situation:• Dietary supplements (amino acids, glucose, vitamins, etc.)Toxic substances in the diet (protection, color of food and other items)The cruel crops used to improve their nutritional value (pesticides, pesticides, herbicides, etc.) used agricultural chemicals.• toxins (heavy metals, other items)Toxicity of the intestine with fermentation of food and powder powder• drugs and drugsTo protect the body from external molecules, the first element of liver protection and the first element, which can act as a selected filter, as most compounds are given by the gastrointestinal path and prepared by the portal neurons. Blood system and liverHepatic arteryOxygenated blood enters the heart through several branches of the aorta, which distribute blood throughout the body. This is a branch of the hepatic artery that supplies oxygenated blood to the liver so that it can perform its normal functions. This is very useful to know.Hepatic blood flow can be summarized as follows:50% by arterial blood flow from the liver• 75% of blood enters the subcutaneous vein-Hepatic veinIn these small blood vessels, called sinuses, oxygenated and nutrient-enriched blood from both the portal vein and the hepatic artery come together to form nutrient- and oxygen-enriched blood. Hepatocytes, or hepatocytes, make up most of the liver mass and perform most of the functions of the organ, receiving nutrients from the bloodstream and secreting waste products. To return blood to the general circulation, the capillaries of the sinuses connect to form the hepatic veins, which return to the heart through the inferior vena cava. The hepatic vein carries blood through:Foods that the body can use in its current form• Foods that are converted in the liver are usable by the body.In fact, the liver is responsible for filtering and removing most toxins from the body. The liver processes 112 liters of blood per minute, or a quarter of the total blood flow in the body. It is clear that this gland is very important. Digestive system and liverGalducts connect the liver to the digestive system. Toxins are removed from the blood by liver cells and secreted into the bile through the bile ducts, which are small tubes or channels in the liver. The hepatic ducts are formed by the bile ducts, which join to form the left and right hepatic arteries. The common hepatic duct, which extends from the liver to the bile duct, is formed by the intersection of these two ducts. The duodenum at the outlet of the stomach is where this tube ends. The duodenum is actually the first part of the small intestine. - Wikipedia Oddi's sphincter, a muscular valve at the end of the gallbladder, controls the flow of bile into the duodenum. The cystic duct is located at the junction of the liver and bile ducts. One needs to move the entire bile from the next meal into the gallbladder, where it will be stored until you are ready to use it to digest fat.Intestinal tubes

Bile entering the intestines consists of:• Fat metabolism requires digestive fluids.The wastes from the liver detoxification are removed from the body and secreted in the feces.Intestine and living systemThe portal vein connects the liver to the intestines and forms an essential link. A malfunction or lack of either of these two organs affects the other.The portal vein carries everything from the digestive tract, including nutrients and toxins, directly to the liver. The amount of toxins that enter the liver depends on the normal functioning of the intestines at that time.? is it rightThe liver is better than any other organ at being able to regenerate some — even much — of its own tissue, unless that tissue is damaged or surgically removed. Removal of 75% of the liver mass does not prevent regeneration of the lost liver tissue. The liver returns to normal weight after about four months. If the intestinal circulation is normal (one stool per day) and the mucous membranes of the intestines that filter waste are in good condition, this value will be lower. When the intestines are not functioning properly, the situation changes. If the digestive system is slow, toxins are easily absorbed and help stay longer in the mucous membranes of the intestines. When excess toxins enter the bloodstream, they can end up in the liver. A person who is severely exhausted has a large amount of debris due to slow bowels.Because toxins and harmful chemicals are in contact with the intestinal lining for a long time, they have a greater chance of damaging the intestinal wall. Micro-lesions form as a result of prolonged exposure and function as open valves through which harmful compounds can enter the bloodstream and be transported to the liver.Toxins can put pressure on the liver, weakening it and making it difficult to produce enough bile. Intestinal transit is further reduced as bile decreases. As a result, when the digestive system slows down, more toxins are absorbed into the bloodstream and transported to the liver. As a result, a vicious circle is created.The liver and intestines play an important role in digestion. RestartIf your ribs are on the right side, you are looking at your liver.Because of its size and importance, it is an important part of our body system. Substances absorbed by food are first sent to this organ, which processes them.Liver: its duties and functionsLiver as a factory. PIERRE VALENTINE MARQUESSO, founder of the first free natural university in Paris in 1935The many functions of the liver can be divided into two general categories:Many body molecules (nutrients) are produced.Removal of toxins and harmful microbes from the body (excretion and protection)? is it right Many functions of the liver produce heat, which raises its temperature. The liver temperature is usually between 102.2 and 105.8 degrees Fahrenheit, which is higher than the rest of the body. When we consume too much, the temperature of the liver rises, which spreads to other parts of our body. This explains why our hands and feet form when we eat too much. Multilateral organizerThe liver performs more than 500 functions. The brain is the only organ that can do many unique things. The liver can do all this at once.? is it rightEtymology reveals the need of the liver for life. In English, "liver" and "life" are very similar words. Liver (leber), which means life in German, has a similar meaning. Sugar storage and blood sugar controlGlucose, sugar, is the main source of energy for cells. The liver converts glucose into glycogen to compensate for the irregular supply of glucose caused by the intervals between meals. To ensure a sufficient amount of this substance in the blood, the liver stores it in its tissues. When blood glucose levels decrease, the liver releases this glucose into the bloodstream to keep the body's blood sugar at a normal level. Without the liver, we would have no energy.If we don't consume enough carbohydrates to convert to glycogen, the liver will make carbohydrates out of fat or protein. However, when we consume large amounts of carbohydrates and our liver glycogen stores are depleted, the excess sugar we consume is converted to fat and stored in the liver. Too much of this fat weakens the liver and prevents it from functioning optimally. Control of concentration and storage of foodsHepatic glycogen is one of the many substances stored in the liver:D-alpha tocopherolsA deficiency in any of the B vitamins, including vitamin B12, can cause harmful anemia.

Some examples of these metals are:When blood levels of these foods decrease, the liver releases more into the bloodstream to restore them to normal levels. If these substances are not available to the liver, deficiency problems can occur. Proteolytic protein productionProteins that help the body are made in the liver from amino acids that enter through the portal vein. Here are some examples:In this form, the proteins in the blood and muscles are called albumin. Two proteins are involved in blood clotting and wound healing: prothrombin and fibrinogen. By doing this, the body can prevent complete bleeding. Port proteins are compounds that the blood uses to transport other molecules. Protein-based supports are used to transport fats, hormones, drugs etc throughout the body. Some of its examples are the transfer of cholesterol by lipoproteins and the transfer of sex hormones in the blood by glycoproteins.Inflammatory proteins (cytokines) initiate a protective inflammatory response of the immune system and allow cells to neutralize harmful invaders. Proteins are not stored in the liver. Produces urea from excess protein and delivers it to the kidneys. The liver has a lot of work to do during this transformation.As the protein overload continues, the liver eventually becomes tired and damaged. Fatty acid metabolismFor example, phospholipids are produced in the liver and are beneficial to the body. It has two options for delivering these chemicals into the body: directly into the bloodstream or stored for later use. Similar to what happens when you eat too much fatty food, fatty liver causes fatty liver when there is too much fat. Fatty liver can be caused by a variety of diseases, including:• Obesity• You have too much fat in your blood• DiabetesGenetic predisposition of man to diseases• Rapid weight lossSome drugs have unwanted side effects. ? is it right What is this, delicious food? Gourmets and feeders eat foie gras, which is prepared from the liver of geese, which becomes fat. In fact, this delicacy is prepared from diseased liver.Detoxification and blood purificationVarious toxins, including metabolic wastes and wastes, are carried through the body through the bloodstream. Filtering these toxins from the blood through the liver forces them out of the body. Bile dilutes substances so that they can be secreted from the body through the intestines. Protection and destruction of dangerous factorsThanks to special cells called Kupffer cells, the liver destroys pathogenic microorganisms, toxic compounds, carcinogens, cancer cells and other harmful organisms. Only the liver can do that. Hepatic functionsWhen the liver is functioning well, the liver protection mechanisms are most effective.A better understanding of the many functions of the liver will help you better understand its role in your health and how you can help it. Blood purificationThere are many diseases that result from the accumulation of toxins and harmful chemicals in the cells and tissues of the body, and blood purification is an important part of this pr ocess.These toxins and hazardous chemicals can cause significant damage if left unchecked. They are:Bal blood increases blood and prevents blood flow (cardiovascular disease)Focus on the joints (arthritis, rheumatism)Asthma can cause respiratory obstacles (bronchitis, colds, asthma, etc.)S kin is soaked in water (acne, eczema and other skin disorders)Or organize groups B or organize (eg Renal or Gallstone)In tissues accumulated as fat reserves (cellulite, obesity)Change cell activity (cancer)Remove the main blocks of liver construction, liver cells, poisoning. In addition to cabbage cells responsible for the destruction of certain infections or other toxins dangerous for the integrity of the body, most liver cells form. HepatocytesThousands of sinus capillaries leave the portal vein and pass through the liver. Each sinusoidal capillary is surrounded by hepatocytes, which form a layer covering the entire length of these vessels. Small "windows" in the walls of these capillaries allow toxins to leave the bloodstream and reach the liver cells. Hepatocytes and capillaries meet in the perisynusoidal space between them. For centuries it was known as dis. This area is full of hepatocyte microvilli that take sinusoidal elements for their own use. Liver cells are called hepatocytesThere are many sources of toxins and harmful chemicals that reach the liver cells. It's your choice. poisonsLoss of protein (urea)Fatty waste (cholesterol, saturated fatty acids)Toxins of intestinal fermentation and putrefaction (indole, box, etc.)Wastes containing carbohydrates (acids, coagulants, etc.)Mineral wastes (sodium, chlorine, potassium, etc.)Hormones are wasted.There are two types of cell bodies: (eg red blood cells)

Hazardous substances• Alcohol• Drugs• antibioticsAccumulation of pollution of toxic heavy metals• Colors and additions to food• Pesticides•

TobaccoLiver cells are constantly involved in the process of blood purification. Due to blood pressure passing through the kidney filter, the kidneys are passively passive, and liver poisoning and harmful compounds are active and their characteristics. To neutralize and deactivate them, in other words, they can be removed without damaging other parts of the body by neutralization .WARNING!Alcohol is not a food, but a poison that the body tries to neutralize to get rid of it. In this situation, the liver is important because it neutralizes 95% of the alcohol consumed. Even if you drink only "a little", your liver still works hard. Every day for one year, you drink 12% alcohol, which equates to 15 liters. How much do you drink in a year? There are two stages in this process of transformation and neutralization.1 phase of the project At this stage, hazardous compounds are converted by several methods:Materials oxidize when in contact with oxygen.• Oxygenation: the substance reduces oxygen. Hydrolysis: Water dilutes the chemical and causes it to break down.Enzymes in liver cells are responsible for these chemical changes. Cytochrome P450 oxidase is one of the most prominent enzymes.second phaseAt this stage, hazardous chemicals are neutralized and deactivated. In this case, the toxic or dangerous chemical is combined with another molecule that has the right properties to neutralize the negative effects, a process known as conjugation. The most common molecule involved in the conjugation process is glucuronic acid. Hepatocytes then neutralize toxins and toxic chemicals along with other components to form bile.Defend yourself and destroy the attackersIn addition, the liver has other specialized cells to fight external and internal attacks that threaten the physical integrity of the body, which is a major challenge for the liver's hepatocytes. As you may have heard, these are Kupffer cells.This is very useful to know. Division of liver cells:80% of liver cells20% Kupffer cellsEgg cellsUnlike liver cells, Kupffer cells are not immobile, but migrate. Because of their location in the capillaries of the sinuses, they are literally submerged in the blood entering the liver. CFber cellsAll risks that have not been neutralized and removed from liver cells can be large macrophages that are large (macrophages) and have the ability to swallow and digest (flat). In the most harmful compounds:Dead or damaged cellsMetastatic cellsDigestion's bad proteins from• bacteria• virusesNetworks carrying disease (AMIB, Plasmodium malaria and more)Yeast (applicant alpians)• Drugs• undesirable chemicals (herbicides, pesticides, antioxidants, protection, etc.)The material created in the labCancer -Creation of Cancer•

THE CIRCULAR SYSTEM 39

DrugsRoll rock music 'n'Pollution that releases harmful chemicals in conditions that throwIt is very useful to know. WARNING! Alien proteins of life! As for proteins, every living human has a unique sequence of amino acids, which is determined by its genetic code. The immune system can distinguish between the body's natural and foreign proteins and recognizes proteins found in bacteria, toxins, plant tissues and other harmful substances as foreign. When we consume proteins (such as those found in fish or meat), the animal meat is broken down by the body into "other proteins" rather than individual proteins.

This is very useful to know.The number of hepatotoxic drugs (destroying liver cells) has increased. This is due to the introduction of new compounds, as well as the delayed detection of hepatotoxicity by previous drugs. Currently, more than 600 drugs are suspected of hepatotoxicity.Doctor of Medical Sciences, Liver Pathologist: Dominique Bessar, Doctor of Medical Sciences,Pathogens are "digested" by Kupffer cells with the help of enzymes. Depending on whether the invader is a living organism (microbe or cell) or harmful (molecular or chemical), it is killed or destroyed. As in both cases, the pathogen is reduced to harmless particles. With the help of this method, Kupffer cells remove all harmful substances from the blood.Kupffer cells can do a lot, but like any other worker, they need time to digest and heal. As in situations where a person is under the influence of various drugs and / or alcohol, his ability to work deteriorates when he is too tired. They catch intruders less and don't confuse them just so they don't get rid of them. As a result, harmful compounds bypass them and enter the body at a deeper level.Imm une system and Kupffer cellsFor example, bone marrow, brain and spleen contain macrophages. They are part of the immune system that protects the body from (its own) and the outside world (microbes, cancer cells, toxins, etc.). Despite the fact that Kupffer cells make up 80-90% of resident macrophages in the body, they do not differ from other macrophages in other organs. Thanks to their number, they have earned a well-deserved reputation as capable defenders. Notice that the huge size of the liver is already known, and these cells make up the bulk of it! The "secret weapon" of the liver is the Kupffer cells, which protect the body from toxins. ? is it right As for harmful microbes, bacteria, viruses and yeast are all in the same family, but the liver can destroy them. Your body has other systems that help fight germs in addition to your immune system. The liver is one of them. Food, drugs, poisons, toxins and other by-products of the digestive tract meet the macrophages of the liver as the first line of defense. While the liver is functioning properly, these dangerous compounds cannot enter the body and accumulate in the landfill. Instead, they are removed before they have a chance to do so. However, when the liver is overloaded and compromised, it enters the bloodstream and then into the tissues. Anti-inflammatory macrophages are then activated to prevent cell breakdown and disease progression. The amount of poison they receive determines whether their efforts will pay off. Digestion of fats requires the production of bile. Galducts collect bile secreted by hepatocytes in the liver. Bile enters the gallbladder and intestines through the hepatic duct, which consists of a series of small ducts. Gaul performs two functions. Removal of toxic and harmful chemicals requires constant secretion and regular excretion into the large intestine. In the small intestine, it helps digest and absorb lipids (fats), which must be excreted periodically (with each meal). The gallbladder makes it possible to achieve these two seemingly incompatible goals. Toxins are removed from the body through the liver and gallbladder channels, which continuously transport bile from the liver directly to the intestines. On the other hand, the gallbladder can store a certain amount of bile and ensure its regular digestion.r oosterEvery day, the liver produces about 1 liter of bile. A liquid with an alkaline pH of transparent and viscous consistency (7.6-8.6). The color of the bile is yellow, its taste is bitter. Sometimes bitter and angry people are called "bile." The concentration of bile in the gallbladder is higher than that of bile which enters the small intestine directly. This bile is also olive green in color. Bile contains the following components:•

DETOXIFYING YOUR BODY

WaterIn addition, gall salts. • Bilirubin• Cholesterol• LecithinMany kinds of mineralsThe emulsifying action of galsals allows pancreatic lipase to completely digest lipids, dividing fat molecules into water droplets. Fat-soluble vitamins such as vitamins A, B1, B2, B3, B5, B6, B12 and omega-3 and omega-6 are easily absorbed when galsals are used to form lipids. If the liver is insufficient, fat-soluble vitamins are not well absorbed, developing deficiency diseases, which leads to deterioration of overall health.Lack of gallstones in the gallbladder can cause the formation of gallstones, resulting in less cholesterol secreted in the bile. Hemoglobin is divided into bilirubin, a gal pigment. These are wastes that need to be removed from the body. The characteristic yellowish-brown color is due to this pigment. The gallbladder becomes blocked to the point that bilirubin can no longer enter the intestines and discolors the stool, while the bilirubin enters the bloodstream and yellows the skin and whites of the eyes and the urinary mahogany. Despite its main role as a nutrient for the body, cholesterol can be dangerous when present at high levels. If necessary, the liver uses bile to remove cholesterol. Cholesterol cannot be suspended in water because it is insoluble. Thanks to the action of gall salts and lecithin, it is able to maintain a suspended state in the bile. Lack of these other chemicals can cause cholesterol particles to deposit (individually and in groups) and form gallstones.Lecithin as an emulsifier promotes the solubility of lipids. As a result, the possibility of their deposition in blood vessels decreases. In fact, lecithin helps lower cholesterol.

TipsLecithin granules and capsules are available for purchase. The recommended daily dose is

2 to 4 teaspoons a day in the form of granules. Granular lecithin can be added to food or dissolved in beverages. "Because capsule content varies from manufacturer to manufacturer, the dosage recommendations provided by the manufacturer are the most reliable source of information. How does the gallbladder work? The gallbladder stores bile for use in digestion. In the duodenum, receptors are activated when fat is found in the food you eat. To do this, the gallbladder receives information from these receptors that transmit nerve and hormonal stimuli to the gland. Each game consists of three stages: The gallbladder empties during meals. The gallbladder contracts three or four times when it senses that lipids have entered the duodenum. The force of these contractions pushes bile out of the cyst duct into the bile duct. After eating, the gallbladder sends its contents into the intestines

to aid in digestion. The gallbladder is empty while the liver continues to produce bile, which is sent directly to the intestines to aid in digestion. To facilitate digestion, the gallbladder should be filled between meals. In this "fasting" state, the intestine does not need bile to break down the food from the previous meal, which has traveled a long way through the digestive tract.? is it rightWhen the gallbladder is filled with stones and cannot be stored and released, surgery to remove the gallbladder is necessary. Further digestion requires bile, which is constantly secreted by the liver. To compensate for the low level of bile, it is better to eat often and in small portions, and also to limit the consumption of fats. Oddi's sphincter, the valve that regulates the flow of bile and pancreatic juice, closes to fill the gallbladder. Oddi's sphincter prevents bile from the liver from entering the intestines, so no more bile is produced.

After returning to the bile and cyst ducts, the gallbladder begins to collect it. The gallbladder stores bile, releasing some of the water to save space in the liver. Therefore, the next meal is accompanied by the release of concentrated and highly active bile. Restart• The liver has the ability to perform more than 500 different functions. Its functions include regulating blood sugar and vitamins, producing proteins and lipids, removing toxins from the bloodstream and removing pathogens and other harmful substances. 80% of liver cells are hepatocytes, and the remaining 20% are Kupffer cells. Toxins are eliminated from the body by liver cells. Kupffer cells in the body can neutralize toxins. Bile is a digestive fluid that helps eliminate waste. During feeding, the gallbladder secretes bile. Fats are better absorbed due to their high content. Liver disease Like any other organ, the liver can get sick at any time in its life. Overeating, chemical contamination of food, alcohol, excessive drug use and doping all contribute to the diseases that affect him, but they are only a small part of the overall problem.Lack in the liverLiver failure occurs when the liver, even without disease, is unable to function at an optimal level. It is commonly called "lazy liver" due to its weakness and lack of energy. If the liver is blocked, blood and toxins cannot pass through it freely. Delayed due to violation of the outflow of bile.The degree of laziness of the liver varies from person to person. Any type of liver deficiency can cause many health problems, as excessive environmental toxicity is the starting point of the disease. However, the digestive system suffers above all else. In addition, they are highly visible and easily identifiable.A person with liver failure may not have all of these problems, although at least some people do:Hard-to-digest fats (eggs, cream, fatty foods, etc.)Concerns about the digestive system• Used for nausea• Swollen and heavy stomach. Burp is another word for gas.• Swelling of the tongue. • Bad breath• Loss of appetiteLack of motivation and fatigue• Yellow skin and eyes• Constipation• Gallstone• Skin rash or itching• HemorrhoidsAlthough mild liver failure is not life-threatening, it can have a negative impact on a person's quality of life. Patients with this disease suffer from stomach problems, are constantly tired and unmotivated. Only when the deficiency is severe does the cell landscape begin to rupture and affect other organs.

Chapter Three

The million

Bile is continuously produced by the liver. There are two ways to digest food: first, by consuming it directly in the digestive tract. Another is to keep a part for later use. The reduction in water content means that the gallbladder holds less bile, so it reabsorbs some of the water content, reducing its volume to 97.5%. Obviously, when this happens, the bile has a high concentration of solids. For example, the percentage of galsals increases from 1% to 6%. Thus, hepatic bile differs from cyst bile in that it is 4-5 times more concentrated, viscous and viscous than hepatic bile. Gallbladder bile contains a high concentration of digestive fluids, so increasing its viscosity is beneficial for digestion. Saturation points are close, and at this point chemicals remaining in suspension can precipitate and form gallstones, which can be dangerous. Overeating is the main cause of gallstone formation. Frequent overeating can damage the gallbladder. The color of its walls darkens. During food, the bile in this organ is incompletely released into the intestines. Because the gallbladder retains part of the drug, there is a risk of excessive concentration in the future. In this way, the gallbladder gradually collects stagnant bile. Removal of cholesterol and minerals in it is inevitable. This is what happens when a substance in a liquid solution solidifies and forms a precipitate. Galsals and cholesterol sit at the bottom of the organs after they are dissolved and suspended. Initially, these compounds are separate, but over time they begin to fuse into larger and larger masses. Mucal bile can lead to the formation of small crystals and eventually gallstones, which can reach several inches in size. The gallbladder is not inherently dangerous, but gallstones can cause it to malfunction. Digestive problems occur when the bile needed for digestion does not enter the small intestine in the normal amount. This creates an environment that is particularly vulnerable to infection. Gallstones come from the gallbladder and present the greatest risk. Galducts or cysts (which connect the gallbladder and the main hepatic duct) can become blocked when an object is too large to pass through the gallbladder or cyst. This can cause severe discomfort (hepatic colic) and localized liver infection (hepatitis or hepatitis). This is very useful to know. Gallstone or viscous bile is a precursor to the formation of gallstones that crystallize and crystallize. Gallstones are the result of the accumulation of these particles. Find the cause of the diseaseHepatitis is an inflammation of the liver. 3 severe disorders are those of greater intensity and shorter duration.Hepatitis causes inflammation of liver tissue. Compression of the bile duct interrupts the flow of bile in the digestive tract. Part of the blocked bile accumulates in the liver and reduces the ability of this organ to detoxify. The rest is absorbed by the body and enters the bloodstream. Because it contains various toxins, if it circulates freely in the blood, it will eventually poison the body. The symptoms of hepatitis are clear. The yellow pigment in bile, bilirubin, is the main agent released in the body during illness. includes:The skin and whites of the eyes appear yellow or yellow (from the French word for yellow: jaune).Dark color of urine (the normal yellow color of urine is due to the presence of bilirubin)• Discolored feces (because they do not get the normal bilirubin from the bile entering the intestines)

Hepatitis can be caused by a variety of reasons, including irritation, inflammation, and blockage of the bile ducts. Below is a list of its various forms:There are two types of viral hepatitis: hepatitis A and hepatitis B. Hepatitis caused by poison or medicine is known as toxic hepatitis.Gallstones block the bile and cause mechanical hepatitis. With hemolytic hepatitis (often as a result of the incompatibility of the blood groups of the mother and the child or blood transfusion), the hemoglobin is too undigested.? is it rightMale hepatitis can damage the liver in several ways. An alphabetical system is used to classify the three main categories.• Hepatitis A is transmitted through drinking water or contaminated food (e.g., salad vegetables, green vegetables, fruits, or seafood). In most cases, hepatitis A is a mild course of the disease with a short duration and rapid recovery.• Hepatitis B is spread through blood, so contaminated needles and other equipment can transmit the disease (indling). In addition, it is sexually transmitted. In most cases, there are no major problems in the correction. • Hepatitis C is also transmitted through blood. Hepatitis C is a major problem because it can become a long-term disease. CirrhosisAs a result of frequent and long-term damage to the liver, ulcerative diseases occur. When cirrhosis occurs, the mass of the liver is affected, and it is a dangerous and long-lasting condition. First ulcers appear, and then scarring (fibrosis) as a result of tissue damage. With the progression of chronic liver disease, the regenerative capacity of the liver is sharply impaired. Many fibrous structures are formed that strengthen the liver and slow down cellular metabolism. As a result, the liver is inevitably damaged. Over time, the organ becomes unable to perform many of its functions properly, including protection, detoxification, and gallbladder production.WARNING!Irresponsible lifestyle leads to cirrhosis. Most cases of liver cirrhosis are caused by alcoholism.The appearance of the liver undergoes drastic changes. Instead of being smooth, its surface becomes hard and dark brown in color. It acquires a purple color and becomes very hard to the touch. The word cirrhosis, which means redness in Greek, comes from this color.Poor liver function can lead to a variety of diseases, including Parkinson's disease and Alzheimer's disease. Even organs located far from the liver can be affected by a decrease in liver function. The liver and other affected organs may seem unrelated, but based on geography and the action of toxins at the source of the disease, the relationship is obvious. Liver and mental healthMany common terms indicate that people have often discovered a relationship between the mind and the liver.A person with "excellent liver" has a calm demeanor and is not easily angered. "Liver Lily" refers to one that lacks chivalry (colorless compared to the usual reddish-brown). A person who tends to "spit out their bile" or have poison is said to be "very emotional" and prone to anger. This phrase was used by the ancient Babylonians to encourage a person to calm down: "Let your liver be calm."The word pitta has two different meanings, both of which are incorrect. This word can be used to describe a person who is nervous and anxious about everything, or a person who is impatient and angry. According to anthropologist Dr. Victor Pott, the cause of these two opposite conditions is not too much or too little bile (if bile means you have too much bile), but rather the resorption of bile in the intestines. Most of the bile produced by the liver is secreted by feces, a small amount is absorbed by the intestinal mucosa. According to Dr. Pat, when there is too much regeneration, our skin burns and blisters. When it is too weak, we feel lethargic, indifferent and angry. The result is the same in any situation: we feel unpleasant and generally unpleasant.

The Digestive SystemDiseases of the digestive organs are often caused by hepatic failure, which is quite understandable because the liver is directly related to this organ.IndigestibleThe double importance of the liver in the digestive process is known. First, the bile breaks down the lipids into smaller pieces, and then they are digested by the digestive fluids of the pancreas and intestines. If this initial step is not done correctly, it can lead to weight gain, nausea and indigestion. The second role of the liver in the digestive process is to alkalize the digestive bolus, most of the food that passes through the digestive tract from your previous meal. The stomach produces a highly acidic digestive fluid to break down protein. The pH level of the digestive bolus when it leaves the stomach is 2.5. Pancreatic and intestinal juices act only in an alkaline environment, that is, at a pH of 7 or higher in the intestines. For the digestive juices to work properly, they must have the right pH level for the food bolus. The pH of the bile it secretes is between 7.6 and 8.6, making it very alkaline. Bolus desalination of the gastrointestinal tract improves fat digestion in a safe and efficient manner. However, in case of liver disease, this alkaline effect may not be sufficient. Fats are not absorbed properly and cause digestive problems. * 4constipationAccording to most experts, lack of nutrition, lack of exercise and insufficient fluid intake are among the most common causes of constipation. However, liver failure is a common and often overlooked cause. One of the functions of bile is to stimulate intestinal peristalsis, which moves digested food through the intestines. Contractions of the intestinal muscles stimulate food fiber and bile. Therefore, even if there is not enough nutrition in the diet, the production of bile is sufficient for the passage of feces through the intestines. When there is little bile, the intestines slow down. With stagnation and accumulation of partially digested substances, the work of peristaltic muscles becomes difficult. Constipation becomes a problem at this stage.Bile is an important lubricant in the digestive system because it moisturizes and lubricates the feces. Bile makes the intestinal mucosa more slippery than usual and prevents feces from sticking to the mucosa. This indicates that the stool can be easily moved forward. The absence of bacteria causes hard stools and slows down the bowel movement.Blood and its circulationAfter the digestive system, the blood and circulatory system are the most vulnerable to liver dysfunction. Rubbish, which is poorly neutralized and not completely removed from the liver, enters the bloodstream, where it accumulates in the form of deposits on the walls of blood vessels. Below are some of the diseases that can be caused by it. Sick fat levelsWhen we eat fat, it goes straight to our liver. All that remains is converted into cholesterol and triglycerides and secreted by the liver in the form of bile. If the stool contains enough food (whole grain shells, plant fibers from fruits and vegetables), this material is usually secreted in the feces. Cholesterol is excreted from the body by fiber. This is a very good point. Without enough fiber, the body is unable to prevent the reuptake of cholesterol. If you do not consume enough fiber, 90% of cholesterol is reabsorbed in the intestines and sent to the liver.As a result, the liver does not process and remove the returned cholesterol in this way, but distributes it throughout the body. Hypercholesterolemia occurs when excess cholesterol accumulates in the blood and is deposited on the walls of blood vessels. Heart disease occurs as a result of accumulation of fat in the blood. Dietary changes and other treatments, such as regular and intense liver stimulation, exercise, and relaxation, can help lower blood cholesterol.Cholesterol is produced not only from excess fat, but also from excessive consumption of sugar and protein. Diseases of the heart and circulatory systemThere are many different types of cardiovascular disease, but they all stem from the same root cause: accumulation of fat molecules in the blood, making the blood thick or viscous. There are certain chemicals that reduce circulation. Atheromas (fat lumps) form in arteries when deposits form on the walls of the vessels, narrowing their diameter and blocking blood flow. Blood clotting occurs when the blood becomes too thick and slow. Blood clots that form as a result of thrombosis (embolism) can cause heart attacks, strokes, and other illnesses. However, a diet high in "bad" fats and sweets will prevent these excess fat compounds from entering the bloodstream if the liver is not overloaded. Any treatment for heart disease should be aimed at stimulating and cleansing the liver.? is it rightMillions of people use blood thinners to treat liver disease and blood clotting caused by overeating. Anticoagulant prescriptions cost more than a billion dollars a year in the United States.

hemorrhoidsHemorrhoids are a type of varicose vein because they are dilated blood vessels in the anus. They are connected to the portal vein, a large vein that runs into the liver. The portal vein, which carries blood to the liver, becomes blocked when the liver is overloaded. Blood accumulates in the portal vein because it does not move and passes through the liver properly. Another consequence of this stagnant condition is that the veins in the anus swell and dilate.Pressure on the nerves of the anus can also play a role when a person tries to have a bowel. One of the common causes is complicated constipation from liver failure.Therefore, liver resection is the main method of treating hemorrhoids. Migraine and migraine-like symptomsDilation of blood vessels in the brain can cause headaches and migraines, and as a result, the surrounding tissues are compressed. Blood vessels dilate as a defense mechanism in response to irritating and hostile chemicals in the blood. If the liver works well, none of these toxins can enter the brain. Liver dysfunction is the leading cause of many headaches. This is especially true for migraine sufferers, as nausea and vomiting are common side effects of these headaches. WARNING! While the short-term use of painkillers can reduce headache symptoms, their long-term effects are counterproductive and self-defeating because they overload the liver and impair its ability to neutralize irritating molecules. Items not mentioned aboveLiver failure can also affect organs located far away from the liver. Additional functions of the liver include the filtration of starch and colloidal wastes derived from lipids.

Foods that fall into this category include wheat and its by-products, such as bread and pasta. It is normal for the liver to remove these wastes from the bloodstream to be secreted through the bile and from the body. When liver function is impaired, waste products cannot be filtered out of the bloodstream and must be removed from the body through the hepatic vein. Thus they can enter the circulatory system of the body and accumulate in the cells of the body. On the other hand, the body can intelligently protect itself from the accumulation of harmful toxins. Too much toxic load for one organ of excretion (in this example, the liver) can force other organs to excrete it. Toxins that cannot be filtered by the liver are now eliminated through the lungs and sebaceous glands. Due to excess toxins in the body, these organs are overloaded and lead to blockage. Mucous discharge through the respiratory system and acne are common side effects of this disease. Diseases of the lungs and respiratory tract (inflammation of the cold) Lungs, bronchi, and sinuses receive unfiltered waste from the blood through the liver. They should not be in these organs, so it is unusual to see them. This causes inflammation of the mucous membranes, which can be accompanied by fever. The colloidal debris binds to the protective mucus secreted by the membranes to protect them. Colds, sinusitis, bronchitis and some forms of asthma can produce a significant amount of phlegm (heard). Restoring normal liver function is the most important step in long-term recovery from respiratory disease. There are different treatments. When liver function is restored, acceptable waste products no longer enter the airways. acneSebum is a fatty substance secreted by the sebaceous glands of the skin that keeps the skin smooth and soft. Toxins in the skin are similar to toxins that are filtered by the liver, and as mentioned earlier, the sebaceous glands help the liver deal with the accumulation of waste products. Acne occurs when the sebaceous glands are filled with excess dirt and can no longer remove sebum properly. Acne is usually caused by hormonal changes that occur during puberty, although liver disease may also play a role. As a result, liver cleansing is widely recommended as a treatment for acne. Solid partial wasteExamples of such discharges are soft and viscous effluents such as mucus or pimples.They are the exact opposite of a solid, insoluble crystal body test. Uracid crystals that form in the joints and kidney stones are two examples of crystal lesions.Metabolic disorders in the body

As a result of liver dysfunction, toxins in the body can lead to a variety of health problems, including diabetes and obesity.Attacks of hypoglycemiaSome people have frequent episodes of hypoglycemia (low blood sugar) for no apparent reason. They experience a rapid loss of energy and strength, as well as weakening fatigue with frequent fainting and dizziness. From time to time they get nervous and tense. Low blood sugar causes fatigue. When this happens, you'll crave sweets like chocolate or candy, and you'll continue to miss them. ? is it right Alcohol, especially when consumed on an empty stomach, can prevent the liver from releasing stored glucose into the bloodstream, leading to low blood sugar and a constant craving for alcohol or sugary foods.Excessive consumption of harmful sugars is the main cause of hypoglycemia, although the liver may also be involved. Normal activity "burns" glucose in the blood. It is reduced in our blood, but we are usually unaware of it. The liver works fast and smart to prevent dangerously low blood sugar from recurring. It does this by releasing glucose, stored as glycogen, into the bloodstream. However, when the liver is depleted, the conversion of glycogen to glucose does not necessarily occur. As a result, blood sugar levels fall below normal, the liver is unable to regulate it, and as a result, people feel tired. Therefore, liver detoxification is the solution. Detoxification and rehabilitation of the pancreas leads to better control of blood sugar. StumbleWeight gain can be caused by a variety of factors, the most common of which is unhealthy liver. In fact, the liver is the first stop for dietary fats before they reach the tissues of the body. Circular fats that are not good for the body, such as trans fats, are usually blocked by the liver. Cholesterol is converted into gal residue, which is secreted in the feces. Because tissues are not supplied with excess fatty acids, weight gain is prevented. This means that excess fat that the body does not need cannot be converted into cholesterol or only in very limited amounts when the liver is weak. Excess fat remains in the bloodstream, and then enters the tissues. Depending on how much fat the liver cannot process and how much fat a person has in their diet, they are formed in this place. As a result, the liver plays an important role in fat metabolism. That's why diets don't always work. Reducing fat intake means that more fat is released from the tissues so that the liver can burn and use as an energy source when dietary restrictions are imposed. On the other hand, diet does not immediately increase the liver's ability to process these excess fats. As a result, dietitians often find that despite their best efforts, their liver refuses to cooperate with their diet. It cannot get rid of excess fat. If you want to lose weight, you need to cleanse the liver so that it fulfills the function of fat met abolism.Protective mechanisms of the bodyThe lack of healthy liver can have such devastating effects on the functioning of the immune system because it allows large amounts of pollutants to pass through it without detoxification. This can cause various health problems.cancerToxic chemicals disrupt the genetic code of cells and cause most cancers. As a result of this process, tumors begin to form. Carcinogenic and mutagenic are terms used to describe the harmful effects of hazardous chemicals on human health. Most often they:Excessive use of alcohol acholl• cyanide and arsenic (from cigarettes)There are many products and drinks containing methylxander, including coffee, tea, soda and chocolate. Tartz with grilled foods (fried coffee)• benzo [a] pirn (meat, fish) in smoked foodIn some cases, chemical food supplementsMyotoxins that grow in enough beans and grainsIn some areas, high levels of drinking water of nitrogen (nitrate), food (especially processed meat) and cosmetics. Accumulation of toxic heavy metals caused by pollution• Some drugsThere is a list of dangerous compounds in the description of the work of the liver, and this list is very comparable. The liver is an important part of the fight against cancer because it neutralizes the mutagenic compounds that form malignant tumors. This is not only a precaution, but also a cure. Thanks to this, the toxic load that promotes tumor growth can be removed from the cell landscape. Despite the enormous potential benefits of liver regenerative therapy, experts have recently agreed that the liver is an important organ in the fight against cancer.Cancer develops as a result of impaired liver function over time. KASPER BLOND, MD, Austria, a famous oncologist, joins the team.Diseases caused by hyperactivity of the immune system- Polyarthritis, lupus and other disorders in which the immune system attacks the body's own cells are common. What's here?Chemical additives, contaminants and other hazardous compounds accumulate in skin tissues, muscles, bones, etc. when a person consumes large amounts of foods containing these substances. The immune system no longer perceives these cells as normal, but as aggressive and dangerous because they are now full of harmful chemicals. Then he turns against them and begins to destroy them.

Normalization of the liver prevents the accumulation of harmful compounds in the cells, which is the best way to fight these disorders.The task of the immune system is to protect the body from damage by eliminating any invaders. The liver acts as a barrier that prevents harmful compounds from entering the body. The immune system is protected by the liver, which works this way. As "liver doctor" Sandra Cabot explains, diseases of the immune system almost always worsen anything that tires or destroys the liver. It all starts with the body. allergyAn allergic reaction occurs when the body's immune system overreacts to a harmless chemical. Non-toxic substances such as pollen, dust, food and insect poison are examples of what this substance can be. However, it is not a dangerous microbe or substance. In people with allergic reactions, histamine is poorly metabolized, and it is more difficult for them to use and secrete it. Allergic reactions occur when the human body is exposed to an allergen by ingestion, skin contact, or inhalation. The immune system perceives it as a threat and activates antibodies to fight it. Antibodies stimulate the body's defense mechanism, releasing histamine (an inflammatory substance). Therefore histamine should be neutralized and removed after use for protective reasons. The liver can do this, but it can also occur in the tissues or in the digestive tract.If histamine is not neutralized and eliminated, it keeps the body in a proinflammatory and hyper-reactive state. Cough and shortness of breath are common symptoms of this disease.Usually, the body is attacked and irritated by toxins, which the liver neutralizes and destroys, causing excessive activity of the immune system. Good liver cleansing is the best treatment for any type of allergy, such as hay fever, asthma, nettles, angioedema (angioedema) or allergies affecting the digestive system.Restar tHepatitis A, B or C, gallstones and cirrhosis are all conditions that affect the liver. People with poor liver function are prone to various health problems: constipation, high cholesterol, cardiovascular problems such as high blood pressure and heart attacks, digestive problems such as headaches, migraines and airway cataracts, low blood sugar, obesity. etc.A guide to liver detoxificationWARNING!It is a prophylactic and therapeutic application of many forms of hepatotoxicity. It is a combination of several brilliant ideas, even if each of them is effective on its own. Any treatment strategy should include dietary changes as a mandatory component. Emptying a bathtub without turning off the water supply is like trying to do so without a drain head. It is a wasted effort. Nutrition modificationBecause our diet is closely related to liver health, liver strength and durability are directly related.When it comes to liver nutrition, there are three things to consider:• Foods we should avoid in our diet.

Some foods deplete the liver resources, damage it or cause stress. It is important to identify these substances so that they do not enter our daily diet. • Useful food for the liver. We have the ability to feed our liver according to it. Nutritional guidelines for maintaining and strengthening this organ can be found here.A diet that helps cleanse the body. The liver benefits from a short-term calorie-restricted diet that allows it to get rid of any toxins it may have accumulated.How safe is liver detoxification? Liver disease can be treated with medication. However, there is no evidence that detox control agents or supplements can reverse liver disease.

Detoxification can damage your liver. The liver damage caused by herbs and supplements is increasing, according to recent research. For example, green tea extract can cause hepatitis. Some diets include coffee enemas, which can cause infection and electrolyte disturbances, which is dangerous. Some other factors to consider are:The materials used by some companies can be dangerous. Many have made false promises about effective treatment of dangerous diseases. Elderly people and people with weak immunity should avoid drinking unpasteurized juices.Drinking too much juice can make kidney disease worse, so it's best to avoid cleansing if you have to. If you have diabetes, you should consult your doctor before starting a new diet.If you fast as part of a detox program, you may feel weak or dizzy, have a headache, or become dehydrated. If you have hepatitis B and your liver is damaged, fasting can make it worse.Yes, cleansing the liver helps the liver recover from alcohol and waste. Detergents have not been shown to remove toxins from the body or improve human health. A non-toxic diet without highly processed foods, including solid fats and processed sugars, will improve your well-being. As for calories, they are pretty bad. For example, milk, gluten, eggs and peanuts can be eliminated from a therapeutic diet if you have allergies or sensitivities. According to medical professionals, liver detoxification is not essential for liver health or performance. There is no evidence that waste or alcohol helps the body detoxify after heavy consumption. Ways to help the liver after excessive alcohol consumptionThe amount of alcohol your liver can handle at one time is strictly limited. When you drink more, your body has to work harder to compensate. Over time, this can lead to ulcers, inflammation or cancer.Doctors recommend no more than one serving of alcohol per day for women and two for men. A drink is a serving of alcohol or 12 ounces of beer.What to avoidMost often, the liver works too hard due to the consumption of certain foods and becomes underused and can even be dangerous. Toxins contained in these products load the liver and force it to excrete them more intensely. With the gradual reduction of his abilities, he ultimately loses the ability to perform his duties. Of products that should be avoided as follows:Oil with hydrogenic fats (with high amounts of saturated fatty acids, usually called trans -fat)• cold pressure oil• mattress and sausage• Smoked food (fish and meat)The sweetest food• Food made of molten oil• fried food• migration• alcohol• black and coffee tea• additional materials in containersTo winYou consume a lot of liver energy to digest bad fats that control the amount of energy in toxicity. Also the normal function of the liver is disturbed as excessive fatty acids (overflowing liver syndrome, fat). For some people, cutting out all sources of fat - animal or vegetable - is a good way to help their liver. However, absolutely not! Removing fat from the diet does not force the gallbladder to release bile into the digestive tract. When bile sits in the gallbladder, it hardens, making gallstones more likely to form. As a result, the muscles of the gallbladder lose tone and the organ is damaged. Supplements of omega-3 and omega-6 fatty acids (omega-3 and omega-6) can have negative effects. If a person stops eating fatty foods, these vitamins are reduced in his diet, which means that some needs that are met in the body will not be fulfilled. Because bile is necessary for the absorption of vitamins and the gallbladder is strained, the body cannot produce enough bile to absorb these n utrients.This means that while it is important to lower bad cholesterol, the body needs good fats to function effectively.

Chapter Four

For my liver

Foods that are suitable for the liver do not overly strain the digestive system, but they do not create toxins that this organ cannot neutralize and eliminate. In addition, the liver benefits from such a diet because it receives various nutrients that help it function properly. This liver friendly diet includes three types of foods. All this is good in itself, but not in itself. However, some should be consumed in moderation because they are more taxed on the liver than others. Due to the high need of the liver, it must be consumed in small quantities. However, they are included in this diet because they provide nutrients like protein that the body and liver need.Eat as much as you want • vegetables, raw and boiledFruits without boiled• nearby beads• herbal tea and water• Unfinished fruit juices and vegetables• spices and plants (other than the pepper -scale)Moderate food• nutsSunflower and linen -bides, pumpkin and other different pumpkins and small grains• carbohydrates: potatoes, rice and chestnuts• Nutritional grains are called whole grains.• Full flour, paste and paste. Smaller sizes are better.• Traveling• FishThis category includes dairy products. • egg• cold oil of plantsExtra sugar -syrup or fructose such as honey, arce -syrup and pear syrupDeveloped fruits and vegetables with Orel, as well as dairy products, eggs and free animals - in front of toxic chemicals (herbicides, pesticides, growth hormones, antibiotics) and their use in the liver and environment. The whole diet is better than food, because most foods are needed. "Light" cooking, e.g. with a minimum fat content (boiled, steamed, baked) is important.Detox foodBy excluding foods harmful to the body and following a healthy diet, the liver will gradually restore its strength and health. However this repair will take some time. You can speed up the liver detoxification process by limiting your diet. * 5In fact, when the digestive process is less stressful, the liver can use its power to remove toxins. It should work with trapped debris, no incoming contaminants. As a result, the decontamination process is significantly accelerated.This type of restricted eating can take many forms if a person limits their caloric intake to less than they are used to. The stricter the diet, the harder it is to keep it physically and mentally.TipsTo maintain a healthy and balanced diet, you should include the following foods in your dietSalad and vegetables make up 2/3 of this portion. carbohydrates and a third of protein.His methodsAnyone can follow the diet I recommend here as it is a bit restrictive. For one to three days, a person eats nothing but vegetables and fruits. Vegetables can be eaten raw, cooked or even squeezed out of juice. Another option is to prepare vegetable soup yourself. Vegetables are best steamed or boiled (without oil). Fruits can be eaten fresh, cooked or squeezed from juice. If you want, you can add fruit juice, but you can't add sugar to them. During a digestive holiday, the liver can remove impurities. If on the first day you feel great, happy and without signs of fatigue, you should continue this diet on the second and third day. Supplementing this diet with herbs, a heat pad or the liver stimulation methods discussed in Chapter 7 can make it more successful.This treatment can be repeated once or twice over several months.

How vitamins helpThe liver needs enough nutrients to function optimally. Vitamins and trace elements are necessary for the action of many enzymes that carry out biological reactions. This requirement becomes more important when toxin levels are high and toxic compounds are particularly aggressive (see Chapter 3 for more information). A rich source of vitamins and amino acids is needed to restore liver cells and Kupffer cells and increase their resistance to foreign chemicals. Food sources of food may not be enough for a sluggish or damaged liver because they do not reach them quickly enough. It should also be noted that the nutritional needs of blocked or dysfunctional liver are much higher. Natural food, a rich source of vitamins, minerals, trace elements and amino acids, is an easily digestible resource to provide the liver with the additional nutrients it needs today.According to research, sulfur-containing amino acids such as methionine and B vitamins are the most important nutrients for the liver. Most of these compounds in natural dietary supplements such as• Used in bred yeastWheat• Bee HoneyWarningPeople with a candidate or yeast infection should prevent using feces, because they can exacerbate their symptoms.Beer used in the production of yeastVegetable juices are therefore very small, seven billion to produce one gram of yeast seven billion. They thrive on the nutrient-rich supplement. Germinated barley and hops are often used to develop a brewer. Methionine is one of the 50% amino acids of a brewer. This food is also rich in B vitamins. There is no better source of B vitamins than brewing yeast and wheat germ. Many foods contain no more than one or two of the twelve B vitamins. Because they work together, the vitamins in brewing are very useful because they all contribute to each other. Beer yeast can be taken in the form of a liquid, tablets or powder. Liquid yeast is more effective than dry yeast because it contains live yeast. dose You can sprinkle the powder on food or add it to a salad or yogurt garment to enjoy its benefits. You can also make a smoothie out of it or mix it with water, fruit or vegetable juice. Be sure to follow the dosing instructions that come with your tablet, as tablet sizes and dosages vary greatly from manufacturer to manufacturer. Follow the fluid manufacturer's instructions. Depending on the severity of the deficiency, treatment should last at least two months. It is recommended to repeat the treatment once a year or every two years. Germination of wheat seeds Like the germ of the future wheat plant, the wheat germ is rich in healthy fats and other nutrients because it contains all the substances necessary for the initial growth of the plant. It has a high concentration of twelve B vitamins. Although it has a lower B content than the brewer, it is an attractive food ingredient due to its sweet taste. In addition, wheat germ is a good source of vitamin E, which helps protect and repair the liver. Wheat germ is a golden and somewhat sticky particle. doseTo make cereals, you can mix everything from water to fruit juice, cereal, yogurt, salad dressing and v egetables.The recommended daily intake is 3 to 4 teaspoons of perc, which is 50 grams. People who are sensitive to wheat germ are advised not to consume more than one to two teaspoons of cereal or brewer per day. After two or three months, if necessary, the treatment should be repeated. TipsWheat seeds (1 tablespoon per day) can be germinated in a sprinkler or in a tray, where one buys wheat sprouts. You can consume both germinated seeds and original seeds within three to five days. Bee pollenThe male seed of flowering plants is bee pollen. It looks like gold dust on a flower. Most bees are known to collect honey, which they use to make honey. Although a typical colony produces more than 100 pounds of pollen per season, it produces only half as much honey. Bees depend on pollen as a source of protein and amino acids, as it contains 40% protein.

Of the eight essential amino acids found in pollen, methionine is present in very high concentrations compared to the others. The content of methionine in 100 grams of pollen is 3.5 grams. Methionine makes bee pollen an effective liver cleanser.? is it rightPure methionine is available as a dietary supplement in tablet form. Cysteine, a precursor of glutathione, is produced when our bodies digest and absorb it, and is a powerful liver detoxifier.Dietary supplement "Methionine" is produced in various forms. As the content of gel capsules varies, it is important to follow the dosing instructions on the package.dosePollen is found in the form of small balls or granules on the legs of bees. The recommended daily dose is 2 to 3 teaspoons. As a result, you can start with a low dose and keep it for the time being. Those who can tolerate the taste, pollen pellets should be chewed completely and then mixed with a large amount of saliva. The rest of us (most of us) can drink it straight or add it to our diet with juice or food. The recommended duration of treatment is from one to three months.sulfideSulfur has long been used to treat liver disease. Harmful effects of sulfur on the liver have been revealed in recent studies.From: Sulfur is good for the liverAs a result, hepatocytes produce more bile. If liver cells do not absorb enough sulfur, the liver's ability to filter toxins and harmful chemicals decreases. On the other hand, if they get enough sulfur, they work well, and adding sulfur increases their efficiency. Detox enzymes are activated. Every biochemical change our body needs to function and cleanse itself occurs with the help of enzymes. If these people get a chance to inspire, a great job can be done. The first onset of liver enzymes is often caused by sulfur. Without sulfur, the metabolic changes necessary to neutralize and eliminate toxins may be absent or insufficient.Removes heavy metals from the environment. Such metals as lead, mercury and cadmium are toxic to the human body. Thanks to sulfur, the liver neutralizes its harmful effects. Through this process of neutralization, toxic compounds are removed from our body, but it also helps to remove them from the tissues and ultimately from our body.Along with methionine, cysteine, taurine and homocysteine, it is one of the four essential amino acids for liver detoxification and regeneration. Using sulfuric amino acids, it is possible to neutralize and remove hazardous compounds.Increases liver oxygenation. Like other cells in the body, liver cells need oxygen to function properly. Among these antioxidants, sulfur is an important food. Products with a positive sulfur contentSuccinic acid can be found in a variety of foods. Defects of this mineral are very rare. On the other hand, increasing sulfur content in the liver improves liver function and promotes detoxification.Foods rich in sulfur can be found in the list below. Mineral water with sulfurSulfur-rich mineral water is good for the liver because of its ability to stimulate the liver. Drink up to 1.5 liters of these fluids daily as a food drink and between meals to help detoxify the liver. The course of treatment usually lasts one to two months. Sulfur is a rare elementSulfur is a rare element. In this form, the sulfur content is significantly reduced. So we have a distribution not in terms of quantity, but in terms of quality. Consumption of sulfur as a rare element not only helps to detoxify the liver by acting as a catalyst for sulfur-containing enzymes, but also increases the absorption of sulfur foods and drinking water in the body. Sulfur is one of the rare elements in the treatment. A dosing device or measuring spoon is usually attached to a small container that contains a liquid. A tablespoon a day is a typical dose. To facilitate absorption, drink on an empty stomach in the morning before breakfast. For best results, place under the tongue for a minute before swallowing. As a result, the whole body can access it immediately. TipsOne teaspoon of liquid trace element sulfur should be taken in the morning, without food or water. Hold the food under your tongue for a minute before swallowing. To control the response of the liver to taking sulfur as a trace element, treatment should be started with a dose every three days. Start once a week and gradually increase the frequency to once or twice a day. If your reaction is severe, stop consuming the trace and replace it with sulfur-rich foods or beverages. A full course of treatment can last from two to four months. In the region of Pay attention to liver fatigue when consuming lipids, sugar and alcohol. • Eat a diet rich in fruits and vegetables that improve liver function. • The nutrients needed by the liver are great. Among the best supplements are brewer's yeast, wheat germ and bee pollen. • Sulfur helps cleanse the liver. Some foods, mineral water and trace elements are ways to get your sulfur intake up. Sources of medicinal plants for liver health Phytotherapy is one of the most effective methods to improve liver function. Medicinal herbs used to cleanse the liver are called "liver herbs" or "liver filters".

Chapter Five

Hepatic plant

Performance of hepatic floraLiver flora has three modes of action:Actions of choleraThese plants stimulate hepatocytes to produce more bile. Doubling the production of bile is a wonderful effect that not only improves digestion, but also helps rid the body of toxic compounds and impurities. Among the common choleretic herbs are artichoke, flatbread, dandelion, dandelion root, milfoil, rosemary, gold rod.Gallant actionsAs for increasing gall bladder secretion, these herbs primarily stimulate the gall bladder. This increases the amount of bile available for digestion and elimination of toxins. As a result, the formation of the gallbladder is significantly reduced. Common weeds include artichoke, bold (capsicum leaves), common barberry, common sedum (a type of fern), and black blessing.Take precautionsLiver cells are protected from these plants. To protect the body from harmful chemicals, liver cells must neutralize them. However, these toxic compounds attack liver cells. Fortunately, nature produces liver protection plants that protect against such attacks.They behave as follows:• By increasing the resistance of the membrane, they prevent the penetration of harmful chemicals into the liver cells. Alcohol, hepatitis virus and other harmful chemicals usually do not enter liver cells. Instead, they are neutralized in the perisinusoidal region (also known as the disc space). On the other hand, some toxic compounds can damage the cell membrane and enter the cell due to its aggressive nature. As a result, liver cells are unable to perform their functions or a large number of liver cells are damaged and die. Herbs that protect the liver are used to prevent or reduce it. Due to the increased synthesis of molecules and enzymes needed by the liver, toxic chemicals are eliminated. Thanks to the increased speed and efficiency of neutralization of these compounds, the liver is protected against their potentially harmful effects. • They stimulate the production of proteins necessary for the repair and regeneration of damaged cells, thus speeding up the process.• They promote cell exchange and keep the liver in optimal working condition. Grass, chrysanthemum, desmodium are some of the best protective plants for the liver (or tick clover).Liver protection herbs should be used in conjunction with a healthy diet and regular exercise for people with liver damage due to medications, drugs, or excessive alcohol use. Anti-cholera, cholera, and anti-hepatic properties are found in various amounts in each plant. The plant always has both choleretic and astringent properties, but one is more important than the other. Only some herbs have a hepatoprotective effect. We know only a few.Do sing with hepatic flora: a quick guideFor a wide and extensive effect on the liver, herbs for the liver are taken three times a day before meals. Three times a day it will stimulate and sustain. With such frequent consumption, the liver will be saved over time. He becomes stronger, returns to his normal state and begins to work more inten sely.Duration of treatmentOverloading the liver with waste and subsequent weakness is a lengthy process. A few days of treatment cannot correct years of constant toxicity. The positive effect of the drug can be seen after a few days, but for a significant effect, the treatment should last two to three months. You can rest for one to two months before starting treatment again. The liver should be kept in good condition for one or two cycles a year. Tips and recommendationsStart with a six-week course of treatment. For more specialized livers, change the flora every two weeks. Over time, you will learn which herbs work best for you.

doseRecommended doses for hepatic flora are based on average values, although each person's response will be different. The average dose is too low for some people, but too high for others. It's important to take only what you need to get the job done, but it can become a burden. Liver flora does not affect the liver. Conversely, the increase in gall production caused by this plant has a laxative effect on the intestines. The feces become more liquid, and its outflow occurs two or three times a day. As a result, the ideal dose without excessive laxative effect on the patient is higher. To find the right dose for you, start with a smaller dose than usual and continue until you feel a mild laxative effect.Eleven herbs that effectively cleanse the liverBecause the action of each of these herbs is significantly different, it is better to use different types for long-term treatment. In addition, this ensures that the body does not get used to the plant and does not react to its presence.Tips and recommendationsTo prepare mother tincture, it is necessary to soak plant raw materials with alcohol in the correct ratio of 10:90. You can buy herbal teas with "liver bladder" or "liver" properties, which are made with a combination of herbs that complement the properties of the liver. A local herbalist or health food specialist can give expert advice. Cleansing the liver with these nine herbs is very effective .Artichoke - plant (Cynara scolymus).The leaves of the flower, not the bud, are used for healing. They are known as liver cleansers because of their ability to stimulate bile production in a mild state. Artichoke leaves are especially useful for young and old people. They also have a small diuretic effect.For infusion, use 5 tablespoons of leaves per liter of water, infuse for ten minutes and drink three glasses a day. This is a strong dry mix.Take one or two gel capsules three times a day. Take 20-30 drops of uterine tincture three times a day.Dairy plant (Cylipum marianum)This plant belongs to the thistle family. It has purple flowers and prickly leaves. Recently, silymarin, a chemical found in milk thistle seeds, has been shown to have liver-protective properties, which is why the leaves are widely used. Drink three cups of brewed tea daily and use one to two teaspoons of this herb in each cup. Take one or two gel capsules three times a day. 20-30 drops of flu are taken three times a day. Amorphophallus sp. (American chrysanthemum) A herb-like plant traditionally used in South America for liver detoxification has recently been found to have liver protective properties. 5 teaspoons per 34 liters of water, boil slowly for ten minutes and drink three times a day. Take one or two gel capsules three times a day. Take 30-50 drops of mother tincture three times a day. Dandelion (Taraxacum officinale) The bright yellow flowers of this popular shrub adorn meadows and pastures. Dent de lion (pronounced Don de Leon) is French for "lion's tooth", referring to the long, fragrant leaves of the plant. Many herbalists believe that this herb is one of the best herbs to maintain liver function because it increases both the production and excretion of gallstones. Dandelions are a great addition to any salad and are very nutritious.

Soak a handful of dried leaves and roots in a liter of boiling water for 10 minutes. Drink three glasses of this tea daily. Take one or two gel capsules three times a day.Take 30-50 drops of mother tincture three times a day. Desmodium is the name of the plant (Desmodium attensense).Desmodium, known for its hepatoprotective and hepatic regulatory properties, is a creeping plant of the legume family found in humid tropical climates.Boil 10 ounces of water, add 1 tablespoon of the dried herb and shake for ten minutes. Drink three glasses of this tea daily.Take 30-50 drops of mother tincture three times a day. Fumaria officinalisThe floral notes of this plant, which is popularly called "hepatitis," are a strong regulator of many liver functions.Drink three glasses a day of an infusion prepared from a large handful of flowers soaked in a liter of water for 10 minutes. Take one or two gel capsules three times a day.10-20 drops of tincture of uterus three times a day. Black radish (Raphanus sativus)Narrow-tipped radishes grow up to 8 inches on each side and can be harvested at any time of the year. Its flesh is white, but unlike other radishes, the skin is black. Radish is known for its sulfur and peppery taste. One of the main benefits of black radish is the stimulation of the gallbladder (cholesterol effect). It is highly recommended to use it in cooking.The manufacturer's instructions recommend consuming 1 to 3 bottles of black radish juice daily. Take one or two gel capsules three times a day.Take 30-40 drops of tincture of uterus three times a day. Let's call it rosemary (Rosmarinus officinalis).Rosemary is a Mediterranean shrub that has strong choleretic and collagenous properties thanks to its small leaves and narrow stems. Rosemary has such a potent effect that it only needs to be used for one month in one treatment. People with nervous disorders should not use rosemary because it has a stimulating and stimulating effect. Recommended for use in cooking. Let the leaves soak for fifteen minutes, then drink two to three cups of the decoction daily.Take one or two gel capsules three times a day. It is recommended to take 20-40 drops of mother tincture three times a day.Flowering plant called Golden twig (Solidago virgaurea).The common name of this plant comes from its yellow floral notes. In late summer, this plant blooms its flowers. Its diuretic and hepatic stimulating properties make it an excellent supplement. Boil water for two minutes, add dry herbal ingredients and infuse for ten minutes. Drink three glasses of this tea daily. Take one or two gel capsules three times a day. 30-40 drops of flu are taken three times a day. Care of a patient with gallstone diseaseAs for gallstones, liver herbs are not just for the liver. Gal-diluting herbs can be used to remove small gallstones from the body that can pass through the cyst duct and gallbladder. Plants with irritant properties promote the secretion of bile. As a result of this drainage process, gallstone sediment and small gallstones are removed, just as the muscles of the gallbladder are strengthened. During digestion, the gallbladder empties more efficiently more efficiently. As a result, foam and small gallstones are removed naturally over time. Black horseradish is medicineBlack radish is a great choice for liver detoxification. The patient uses it in the morning on an empty stomach for up to two months. Mix Thai tincture with lemon juice to make 1 teaspoon (50 drops) of black blessed tincture. Add this mixture to a large glass of water and stir. Lemon is a supporting player in this dish. As a result, the secretion of the liver, stomach and pancreas is stimulated. If you are sensitive to fruit acids, it is best to avoid taking this supplement. Bottles of black blessing juice can replace motherhood of black blessing. The choleretic effect of black blessing is slow and mild. As a result, large gallstones cannot be removed from the gallbladder by the use of this drug. The gallbladder muscles are actually strengthened in a very gentle way. Sludge and small gallstones are removed over time. Dandelion, on the other hand, works and is prescribed in the same way. Squeeze olive oil You can also clean the bladder with olive oil. The gallbladder contracts when fat leaves the stomach and reaches the duodenum. However, this process can be misused by consuming large amounts of fat between meals rather than during meals. If the gallbladder is filled with small gallstones and other gall debris, this process causes them to be irritated and secreted. For a long time, the best lubricant for this job was olive oil. Use only extra virgin olive oil in cooking.

There are two options:• Take 1-2 tablespoons of olive oil in the morning on an empty stomach for ten to fifteen days. Repeat this treatment several times a year. The night before the procedure, eat nothing but vegetables, such as vegetable soup or raw vegetables. Take 6-7 tablespoons of olive oil in the morning before meals. 30 minutes after the oil enters the duodenum, there is an active secretion of bile. Repeat the treatment three times a week or once a month for three months. There is a risk of injury with this method. Consumption of a large amount of oil puts a heavy burden on the digestive system. Add some lemon juice to the oil to make it easier to digest.Reducing the size of gallstonesGallstones that are too large to pass through the cyst and gallbladder pathways to the intestines must be removed surgically. Simply put, they are wider than these pipes. So finding a way to solve gallstones can be a good solution. Once they become "dusty," the bile can easily remove them.Over the years, various medicinal plants have been proposed for this purpose. Among them, we can mention artichoke, bold, birch, nettle, black radish and many other plants. However, their statement on the liquidation of factories should be treated with skepticism. In fact, there has never been any indication that these plants can do that. The positive effects observed after use of these herbs can be attributed to the energetic evacuation of the gallbladder. With large gallstones, the pipelines are cleaned of gallstone and small gallstones. Using heat, exercise and massage to stimulate the liverIn addition to nutrition and herbs, there are external methods to stimulate the liver and ensure its optimal work.hot water tankHot water bottles are a great way to stimulate the liver. The liver is the warmest organ in the body, with a range of 102 to 105.8 degrees Fahrenheit (39 to 41 degrees Celsius). The action of the liver emits a significant amount of heat, so it is used not only to work at such a temperature, but also necessary for its normal functioning. The liver needs heatThe speed with which the liver performs its functions is reduced due to heat loss. This can happen when a person is ill, but it can also be caused by excessive activity, stress, poor diet, nutritional deficiencies or not having enough warm clothes for the weather. When the liver temperature drops, the blood vessels in the liver capillaries narrow. By reducing the diameter of blood vessels, the volume of blood in them also decreases and causes stagnation in blood circulation. It is known that the liver in its natural state is well supplied with blood. It weighs 3.3 pounds dry. Soaked in blood, it can weigh up to 5.5 pounds. That is why almost half of its total weight is blood. Serpentine sinusoidal capillaries transport this blood between liver cells. The lack of blood supply to the liver impedes the cleansing and removal of debris. An increase in blood flow can immediately solve this problem of hypothermia in the hepatic area. This can be done relatively easily and efficiently with a heating pad. A hot water bottle can speed up the metabolism of the liver by raising the temperature of that area. By placing a bag of warm water on the area where this organ is located, you can increase the temperature of the liver. As the capillaries in the liver dilate, more blood flows to the organ, normalizing blood levels. While the heater is in use, it can reach this level. Having regained vigor and strength, the liver returns from its state of inactivity. Detailed instructionsThe liver area is a good place to put the warm water bag in front of the body. It is not necessary to heat the water in the kettle, as the tap water is already quite hot. The heating pad can be used directly or on the skin.Stay there for at least half an hour, if not an hour. Start with ten-minute sessions and work up to thirty to forty-five minutes, staying as still as possible (lying down or sitting). Some movement is allowed, but not so much that the heating pad falls off the target. Use one to three times daily after meals. If you want to do a session immediately after a meal, while sleeping or before going to bed.

Chapter Six

Workouts

Hepatic blood circulation is uniform, strong and abundant, 1 liter per minute of the total body volume of 5 liters. All this blood is necessary for the normal functioning of the liver. When the liver is overpopulated, blood and waste products accumulate in a stagnant state, and in a vicious cycle, decreased blood flow exacerbates the problem, making it difficult for blood flow to keep the flow in the organ. This is possible if the blood flow from the liver does not "drain" the blood below 1 liter per minute. Insufficient pressure impedes the filtration process.Congestion in and around the liver is partially relieved by physical exertion. Exercise generally increases blood flow, and the liver is no exception. WARNING! These exercises should be introduced gradually and done within the limits of your physical abilities, without exaggerating it for the benefit of your health. With two flexion movements, you can massage the liver on the face and increase blood circulation, doing exercises until fatigue. Using flexion exercises for self-massage of the liver These flexion exercises are necessary to remove blood from the liver and gallbladder. Thanks to the contractions caused by these exercises, the free and wasteful blood in these organs is pushed further into the circulatory system. Fresh, oxygenated blood rushes in to fill the hole in the artery. As a result of repeated movements, the liver is repeatedly compressed and deformed. Trunk bending in the middle Consider the standing position at the beginning of the exercise. The hands should be folded behind the head, and the elbows spread to the sides. Flexion and extension of the trunk to the sidesPractice bending to the sides during inhalation and exhalation and alternately bend left and right.• Leaning on the right side, breathe deeply to compress the liver well. Take a short break between each set of 10, 20 or 30 slopes.Coils from head to toe• Sit down early. Put your hands into fists and place them at the base of your neck with your elbows out.• Lean forward until your body meets your knees, keeping your back as flat and straight as possible. Inhale by leaning forward, then exhale while straightening. •Three sets of ten, twenty or thirty inclines a day, with rest between each set. DirectBreathing as a means of improving blood circulationA normally functioning liver circulates an average of five milliliters of blood per minute. If the liver filter is blocked, this is not an option. It is also possible to restore and increase the normal blood circulation of the liver with the help of physical exercises. What is the use of this? In order for your muscles to function properly, you need access to enough oxygen. The body's need for oxygen increases in direct proportion to the intensity of muscle training. To fulfill this need, we breathe more deeply and quickly to get maximum oxygen. Blood flow, which delivers oxygen to the muscles, accelerates in response to increased respiration. Then it is quickly and widely assimilated by the muscles. When you are tired, your heart and lungs work harder, which means more blood flow to and through your liver. Work your thighs, which are the largest muscles in your body, to breathe quickly. Exercise increases the need for oxygen, which increases rapidly. Exercises targeting the hips can double or even triple blood flow to the liver.Examples of various exercises:

crouchPlace your feet slightly wider than the shoulder width apart.Bend your knees to pull your hips through your heels as if you were ready to sit on a chair. Stretch your arms out in front of you for balance.Straighten your legs and return to the forward position, sitting on your heels. If you can, make three sets of ten to twenty curls, depending on your ability.Be sure to rest between sets. You will soon feel short of breath and your blood flow will accelerate faster as you do a squat. • Increase the speed of the squat over time. Another name for running is running.• Keep up the pace until you feel breathless. • After you stop running, do a long, slow jog to normalize your breathing and heart rate.Repeat this several times, alternating between walking and running.

You will get tired faster on an uphill road than on a flat road.cyclingIf you're cycling for 15 to 30 minutes or more, ride at a steady pace (or use an exercise bike). The exertion causes severe shortness of breath and a sudden increase in blood flow through the body, including the liver.Instead, you can do a lot of additional exercises. In fact, any type of intense exercise or sport is done without air. If you choose something you like, you're more likely to stick with it. MassageLiver massageIf the liver is blocked, massaging it can remove the blockage and improve it. However, unlike the intestines, the liver is hidden between the ribs, where it is protected from external shocks. However, this can be achieved by following the boundary of the ribs in the upper abdomen and right thigh. You can directly affect a small portion of the liver by massaging the soft tissues of this area, in other words, "feeling" the liver, slightly soaking the tips of your fingers behind the ribs. It has a wavy effect through the liver. For liver massage, rubbing is used in the defined area. A hard surface makes it easy to get out of bed. Apply circular pressure to the liver area with three long fingers of the left (or right) hand. Friction should be light and shallow at first, but over time it should become more intense. Initially, massage two or three minutes a day, but gradually increase the time to twenty minutes. Foot reflexology: reflex zone massagePlantar reflex zones are areas of skin where a nerve from another organ terminates on the sole of the foot. Each part of the body is related to a specific area of skin on the sole of the foot, called a skin spot. The decrease in the health of the limb as a result of this relationship affects his reflex zone. If the organ is diseased, the area becomes unpleasant to the touch. The severity of the disease that affects the organ indicates the strength of the pain caused by it. Through this link, information can be sent in both directions. Conversely, the organ to which the reflex zone is connected is stimulated by massaging the reflex zone. This technique uses a thumb or knee massage. First, simply rub the reflex area for a few minutes two to three times a day (two to five minutes). Massage can be done for 10 or 20 minutes at a time. Before you start massaging the reaction area, apply some oil or cream to the skin so that your fingertips can slip on the surface and not irritate the skin. The lower part of the right foot has reflex zones for the liver and gallbladder.

Reflex areas of the liverIn real life, the liver can be stimulated in many ways.A temperature of 102 to 106 degrees Fahrenheit is ideal for liver function. Heaters increase the temperature of the liver and stimulate its activity. The liver contracts during chest exercises such as lateral flexions and forward flexions. As a result, blood circulation improves and the work of the liver is stimulated. Reactive areas of the liver on the soles of the feet can be stimulated by direct friction or pressure. Treatment of the liver with internal organsThe intestine can also be used as an indirect access route to the liver. When intestinal transit is normal, toxins in the feces interact briefly with the intestinal mucosa. With severe constipation, the duration of contact with feces increases. Some negative consequences of prolonged contact:• The body absorbs a large amount of pollution. Due to the aggressive nature of the toxins, the intestinal lining is damaged, allowing the toxins to enter the bloodstream and thus be transported to the liver through the portal vein. Reduces intestinal traffic disorders. These negative effects can be reduced by restoring normal bowel circulation, and this can happen a little faster than usual .Toxins are secreted before absorption, so the liver must treat some of them as they pass through the small intestine. Intestinal transit can be accelerated in several ways.LaxativesThis type of laxative is a drug that promotes bowels. Some herbs, including alder alder, golden rain (Cassia fistula), or mallow, can help drain the intestines. These herbs are best used as Thai dyes because of their taste. In this situation, 15 to 50 drops three times a day is enough. Drink some water with it before meals. Buttermilk powder in powder formAnother option is to use milk powder (the liquid that comes from frozen milk) as a mild stool softener (available at most vitamins and grocery stores). 1 tablespoon buttermilk for half a glass of water is recommended. As a healthy snack, drink two to four glasses of water a day before or after meals. Depending on how you feel, you can increase or decrease the number of cups of buttermilk you consume. For best results, follow this program for one to two weeks. * 6Food rich in fiber for weight lossFoods rich in mucilage, such as flaxseed and banana, are rich in fiber and are often used to treat digestive problems. Fecal transit is facilitated by peristalsis caused by the contact of these fibers with water, causing them to swell five to ten times their original size. These two diets complement, not replace, a diet rich in fiber (whole grains, fruits and vegetables). Here is your decision:1 to 3 teaspoons of ground flaxseed per day with food or drink is recommended. Chew them for a few minutes before swallowing. Drink plenty of water later.The recommended dose of psyllium is 2-3 tablespoons of psyllium powder mixed with water a day. Gradually increase it until you find the right dose for you. After taking a plantain, you need to drink plenty of water. Some fruits have laxative propertiesSome fruits significantly accelerate intestinal transit. Regular consumption of these types of fruits helps cleanse the intestines. Two or three plums can be eaten as they are or soaked overnight in a bowl of water. Check the dose to get the desired effect. Two or three dried figs can be eaten as is or rehydrated in a bowl of water overnight. You will have to experiment a bit to find the right size. at workRegular intestines help the liver to function properly.There are several ways to speed up the work of the digestive system and reduce the burden on the liver:• Laxatives• Buttermilk powder• Foods rich in fiber• Fruits with laxative propertiesInstructions for the treatment of the patientThe liver can be treated by a variety of methods. You can determine the best procedure for your situation by trial and error. I will show you four examples of how these treatments differ from each other. Each will contain information about who it affects and how.WARNING!

Each of these methods requires adjustment of the diet. A simple solution is to eliminate the most dangerous foods from your diet (see Foods to eliminate from your diet). In addition, you need to eat healthy liver to reap the benefits of intensive care.Easy work(from several weeks to months)Those who want to do the following are eligible to receive this treatment:• Responsibility for personal health• Learn about the detoxification process• Elimination of congestion in the liver caused by fatty and sweet foods (for example, during a trip or holiday).Liver condition:• A little tense. • Light cleaning required.The liver is stimulated and detoxified. Here's what we do: There are two methods of detoxification.

DETOXIFYING YOUR BODY

Another way you can choose from the list below is to take herbal supplements to treat your liver. Plants used to treat• Congress• Dandelion• radish, blackFollow the instructions of Chapter 6 on the management of your chosen drug.Additional proceduresOver the herbal above methods, explained by one of the following methods to help the liver toxic process:Use a hot water bottle at night (especially for those who are cold))An irregular elementYou get reflexology for five to ten minutes daily. • Vitamins (beer yeast or bee pollen) are great for people who are constantly tired and suffer from a lack of energy.Simple long-term treatment(three and six months)Patients who should receive this treatment include those who fall into one of the following categories:You will always have intestinal problems.• You have difficulty digesting fats and heavy foods. Liver condition::• Density, accumulation• Fatigue and lethargy• Weakeffects:Reduces clogging of the ducts• Performs device functions• Increases liver functionAs part of this treatment, three medicinal plants and two other detoxification methods are consumed consecutively.Medicinal plantsTake a different herbal remedy from the list below each month. Example:• Art shocks in the first month• In the second month of milk• The golden vine blooms in the third month of the year.Chapter 6 of the guidelines describes how to provide treatment. Replace the herb that causes muscle cramps, indigestion or other symptoms of malabsorption with another herb.Additional methods of treatmentTo cleanse the liver, you can use the following herbal remedies along with herbs:1-1.5 liters of sulfur mineral water dailyAs a supplement, you can take bee pollen and / or brewer's yeast. Intermediate treatment.

(a few weeks)Patients who should receive this treatment include those who fall into one of the following categories:Stress and fatigue• Eating too many foods, especially foods with low nutritional value.• Alcohol abuse and stimulants. Hepatic failure:• High trafficStress and fatigueAs a result of a short course of treatment, the liver is significantly cleansed, though not completely.This treatment combines one herb with five different detoxification processes to help cleanse the liver. Medicinal plantsYou have three plants to choose from:• Rosemary• Dandelion• Black radishChapter 6 of the guidelines describes how to provide treatment.Additional methods of treatmentCompletion of herbal treatment with the following drugs will increase its toxicity:Sulfur vegetables should form the main part of your diet. • Use the heater three times a dayUse a sulfur supplement, which is a rare element• Reflexology massage of five to fifteen minutes twice a dayBeer yeast or bee pollen are two choices for dietary supplements.Intense therapy continued(from several weeks to months)Patients who should receive this treatment include those who fall into one of the following categories:There should be constant weakness of the liver. • Common bowel problems.• You have difficulty digesting fats and heavy foods. Hepatic Health:trafficBreak too much loadEffects:Reduces gall pipesLiver increases liver functionLive helps to reproduce the liverThere are five real and real toxic methods to help clean and restore the liver and restore the liver.Plants used to treatCreate this habit to consume one of the herbs under each month. Example:• Dandelion is the flower of the first month.Regular smoking in the second month• Green mung beans - the third month. Chapter 6 of the guidelines describes how to provide treatment.

Note: If your body has trouble digesting the herb (such as cramps, swelling, or other symptoms), switch to another herb. Additional methods of treatmentTo cleanse the liver, you can use the following herbal remedies along with herbs:Sulfur is an unusual elementUse a heater at night.Reflex massage once or twice a day for five to fifteen minutes. Additives (such as brewer or bee pollen) may be required.• Exercises / curvesat workShort or long-term treatment can be chosen according to your specific needs and the condition of your liver. You choose and use a combination of liver stimulation methods (liver herbs, hot water, exercise, massage, etc.). Dietary changes are very important in all these treatments. Initially, avoid highly toxic products.

CPSIA information can be obtained
at www.ICGtesting.com
Printed in the USA
BVHW031354290722
643329BV00015B/928